JASON GYRE

GATEWAYS TO HEALTH

THE FIVE HEALING TIBETANS

SIMPLE EXERCISES FOR REJUVENATION AND HEALTH

WATKINS PUBLISHING

LONDON

613.70 46
G

Distributed in the USA and Canada by
Sterling Publishing Co., Inc.
387 Park Avenue South, New York, NY 10016

This edition published in the UK 2009 by
Watkins Publishing, Sixth Floor, Castle House,
75–76 Wells Street, London W1T 3QH

Conceived, created and designed by Duncan Baird Publishers

1 3 5 7 9 10 8 6 4 2

Designed by Clare Thorpe
Commissioned artwork by Art-4

Printed and bound in Great Britain

Library of Congress Cataloging-in-Publication Data Available

ISBN: 978-1-906787-07-3

www.watkinspublishing.co.uk

For information about custom editions, special sales, premium
and corporate purchases, please contact Sterling Special Sales
Department at 800-805-5489 or specialsales@sterlingpub.com

Contents

Introduction

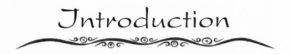

The Five Healing Tibetans were first brought to the attention of the world by Peter Kelder in 1939 in his book, *The Eye of Revelation*. The book describes how a retired British army officer was taught a set of exercises by monks in a remote Tibetan monastery in the Himalayas. After a while the officer noticed that his body looked and felt younger, and he believed that the exercises were instrumental to his rejuvenation. After leaving the monastery, the officer taught the exercises to several people, one of whom was Peter Kelder.

Nobody knows if a brotherhood of Tibetan monks was the original source of the exercises, but what is certain is that the exercises are simple to perform (with practice they can be performed in around ten minutes) and practising them gives you real health benefits.

Specific examples of health benefits that have been attributed to the Five Healing Tibetans are:

weight loss, greater vitality, easing of aches and pains, and better muscle tone.

Take Care

Unless special care is needed for a pre-existing condition, performing the exercises described in this book will be more beneficial to the health than doing no exercise at all. However, please consult your doctor if you have any complaints for which you are receiving ongoing treatment. Particularly if you are suffering from any of the following conditions: duodenal and stomach ulcers, hiatal and inguinal hernias, high blood pressure and spinal problems. It is also advisable to seek medical advice before starting if you are pregnant.

If you are at all concerned, you can try the Preliminary Exercises described before the Five Healing Tibetans (see page 14). Finally, if you want to learn about meditations that may make the Five Healing Tibetans even more effective see page 58.

The Energy Body

One of the reasons why the Five Healing Tibetans are thought to be so effective relates to the theory that all living beings have energy bodies that underlie their physical bodies. Just as certain exercises are good for the physical body, some are good for the energy body. Any exercises that benefit both are said to be particularly effective.

Broadly speaking the energy body contains a central channel and two side channels that are intertwined with it. The side channels switch sides at several points, which are referred to as *chakras*.

The central channel corresponds with the spine and the energy centres have physical correspondences in the endocrine system. This correspondence works both ways: a healthier endocrine system results in more energy for your energy body while a healthier flow of energy through your energy body helps balance the secretions of your endocrine system.

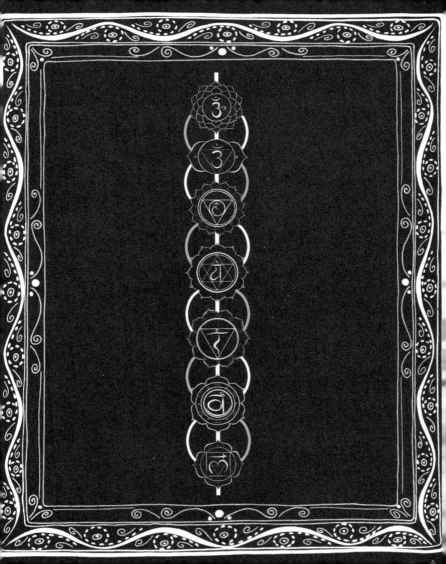

Before you Begin

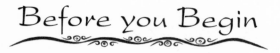

No special preparations are required to perform these exercises. All you need is room to lie down and enough space to stand with your arms outstretched. However, take care that the floor is not too smooth and slippery or too rough and abrasive.

It is best to perform the exercises while wearing a minimum of clothing, so a space that is both private and warm would be ideal. Otherwise you can perform the exercises wearing loose clothing, but make sure that it is not too baggy that it could become tangled.

Take Care

Ideally the exercises should be performed on an empty stomach, since digestion itself can involve a fair amount of work for the body (which is why you might feel sleepy after eating a large meal). In addition, some of the exercises involve movements that may lead to feelings of nausea if performed on a full stomach.

This means that it is probably best to do the exercises when you wake up or just before going to bed. This also has the advantage of reducing the likelihood of interruptions, which could interfere with proper performance of the exercises. When you do the exercises a decision should be based on whether you find the exercises invigorating or relaxing. To some degree this depends on your state of mind, and if you wanted to, you could perform the exercises once upon waking and once before going to bed. However, doing the exercises twice a day is by no means a requirement to gain appreciable benefit from them.

Finally, the first time you perform the exercises be sure to read all the instructions carefully and, until you are confident, review your practice against the instructions afterwards. Otherwise you may not notice any mistakes before they become a habit and are thus more difficult to correct.

Correct Breathing

Breathing is something you do without any need to think about it. As with all activities that are done without thought, you can get into bad habits.

The most important rule of correct breathing is to breathe evenly and deeply with no pause between exhalation, inhalation and exhalation; always breathe through the nose with a minimum of noise. This is best applied through the use of breathing techniques such as diaphragmatic breathing. The key to this is keeping the extent you move your upper chest and lower abdomen similar.

1   Sit upright on a chair with your feet a little distance apart flat on the floor. As you inhale feel your ribs expand, your upper chest and lower abdomen move forward, and your head move back.

2   As you exhale your body returns to its original position: head facing forwards, and back straight.

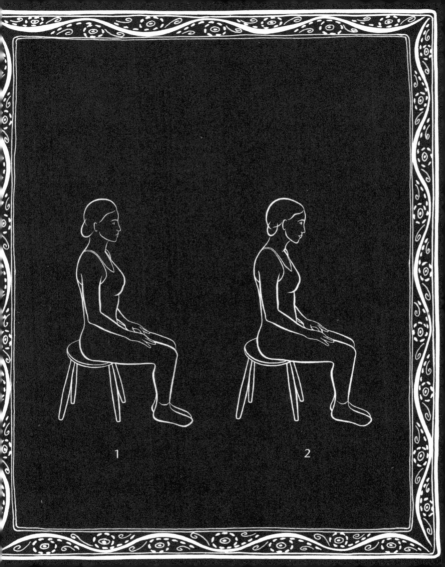

1

2

Proper Posture

These exercises will naturally improve your posture, but the development of proper posture independently of the exercises will help you get the most benefit from them. Another good reason to improve your posture is that bad posture can lead to bad habits in breathing.

The figures on the facing page illustrate how to stand straight and how to sit straight. In the standing posture, imagine a cord suspended from the top of your head that passes through your body to the ground. If you stand correctly the cord should pass through the vertebrae of the neck and the lumbar regions, behind the centre of the hips, and in front of the centre of the knees and the ankles.

In the sitting posture, try to sit against a wall with just the back of your head, your shoulders and your sacrum touching it.

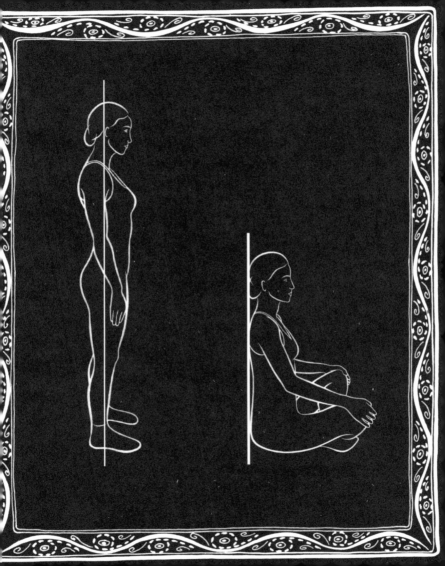

Preliminary Exercises

Some of the exercises in the Five Healing Tibetans involve moving your body in ways you may not be used to. Therefore it is a good idea to begin with the simpler exercises presented in this chapter to gain confidence in your abilities before starting to practise. Although the optimum number of repetitions for the Five Healing Tibetans is 21, for the preparatory exercises start with three repetitions, gradually working your way up to ten repetitions per exercise, by which time you will be ready to begin the full exercises.

Relaxation

The ability to relax fully is fundamental to the practices that provide the spiritual basis for these exercises. In addition, practising relaxation before and after your exercise routine will reduce stress

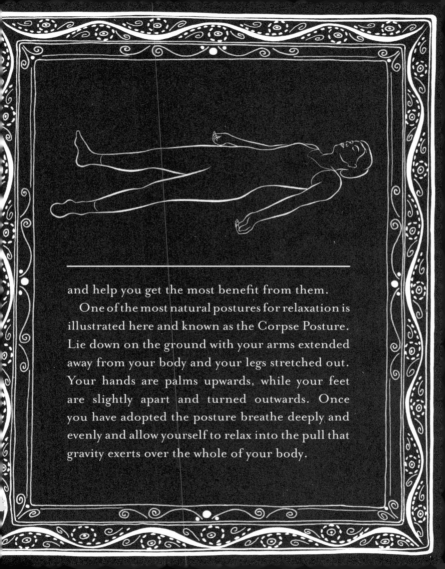

and help you get the most benefit from them.

One of the most natural postures for relaxation is illustrated here and known as the Corpse Posture. Lie down on the ground with your arms extended away from your body and your legs stretched out. Your hands are palms upwards, while your feet are slightly apart and turned outwards. Once you have adopted the posture breathe deeply and evenly and allow yourself to relax into the pull that gravity exerts over the whole of your body.

Neck Exercises

Each exercise begins with you standing or sitting in the correct posture (see page 12).

1   Move your head forward until your chin rests on or near your chest. Lift your head until it is tilted as far back as is comfortable.

2   Keeping your head and neck level, turn your head gradually to your right as far as is comfortable. Hold this position for a few moments. Then, still keeping your head and neck level, turn your head gradually to your left. Hold for a few moments.

3   Keeping your head and neck straight, tilt your head towards your right shoulder (but do not move your right shoulder) as far as is comfortable. Hold this position for a few moments. Then reverse the process and tilt your head towards your left shoulder as far as is comfortable. Hold this position.

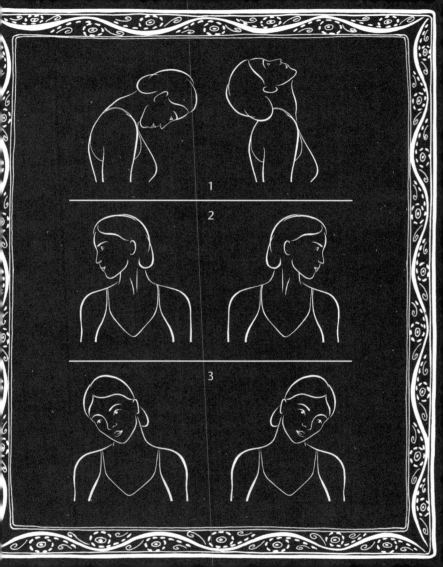

Preparation for Healing Tibetan One

Healing Tibetan One can make you dizzy so this is a good way to start getting used to the sensation.

1   Stand with your feet shoulder-width apart and head straight. Hold your arms outstretched to the side at shoulder height with your palms facing downwards and your fingers and thumbs together.

2   Swing your arms to the right as far as is comfortable, keeping arms outstretched all the while. As you swing to the right, your torso, head and left foot should follow the movement, and your left heel will lift from the floor.

3   Swing back to the left and continue until your arms are as far left as is comfortable. Again, your torso, head and right foot should follow the movement and your right heel will lift from the floor.

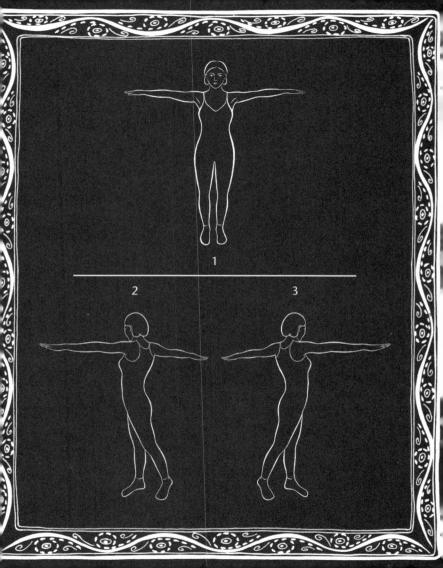

Preparation for Healing Tibetan Two

The next two exercises will help to prepare you for Healing Tibetan Two.

Take Care

Perform this exercise slowly. Be careful not to 'pull' the head forward with your hands; the pull should come from your abdominal muscles.

1   Lie on your back with your knees bent and your feet flat on the ground, shoulder-distance apart. Place your hands behind your head with your elbows slightly lifted. Breathe in without lifting your shoulders.

2   Breathe out, drawing your stomach in and slowly curling the head, neck and top of the shoulders up so that your eye line is between your knees. Your tailbone should be heavy and the front of the hips relaxed. Breathe in as you slowly curl back down.

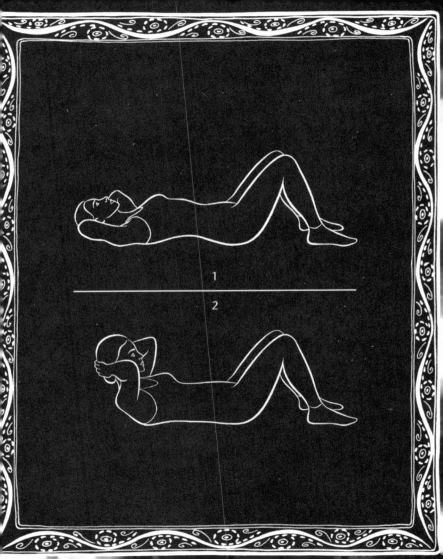

1

2

This exercise will get you used to lifting your legs vertically. Although it is similar to the second exercise of the Five Healing Tibetans, it should not tax the abdominal muscles or the back.

1 Lie on your back with your legs and feet together so the toes point upwards. Place your arms by your sides with the palms facing downwards and keep the fingers and thumb of each hand together.

2 Raise your left leg from the ground until it is completely vertical. Hold this position for a few moments, then lower your left leg back to the ground.

3 Raise your right leg from the ground until it is completely vertical. Hold this position for a few moments. Lower your right leg back to the ground.

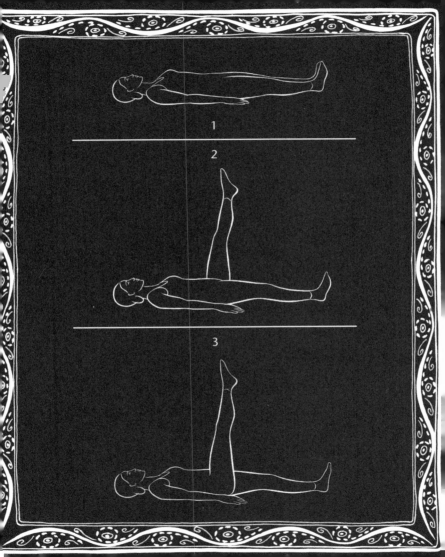

1

2

3

Preparation for Healing Tibetan Three

Stretching the back should be approached with caution, so master this exercise before attempting Healing Tibetan Three.

1   Kneel with your upper legs perpendicular to the floor, legs slightly apart and toes flexed. Keeping your head straight, hold your upper body upright with your arms unbent by your sides.

2   Extend your right arm directly in front of you and reach back with your left arm to touch your left heel. As you reach towards your heel, look down your arm. Restore your upper body to an upright position with your arms by your sides.

3   Extend your left arm directly in front of you and reach back with your right arm to touch your right heel. Return to the upright position with your arms by your sides.

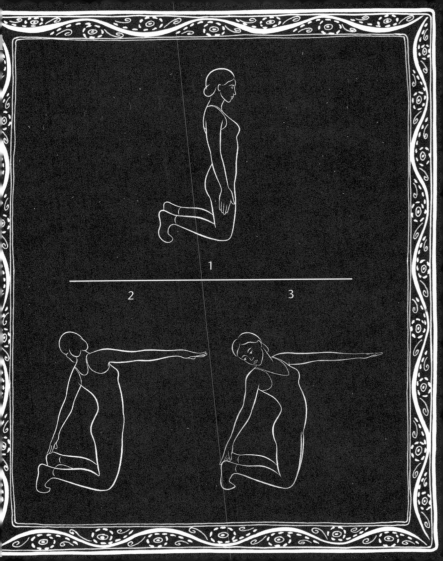

1

2   3

Preparation for Healing Tibetan Four

For strengthening your back and pelvis.

Take Care
The very simplicity of this exercise can lead you to strain yourself, so beware.

1   Lie flat on your back, with your arms straight and palms down, your knees bent and feet flat on the floor, slightly apart.

2   As you breathe in, push your pelvis up a few inches off the floor and hold it for 10 seconds. As you exhale, release and lower your pelvis to its original position.

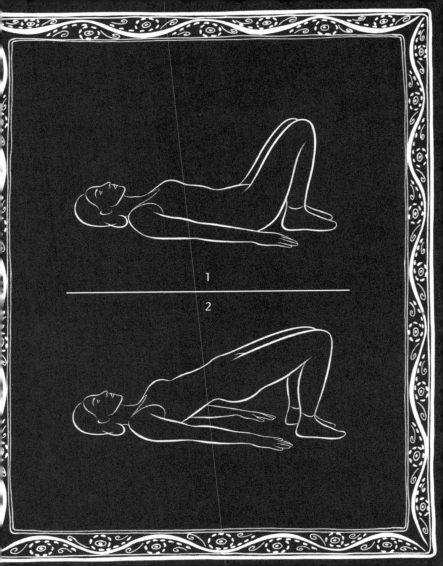

1

2

Preparation for Healing Tibetan Five

The first exercise will help to increase flexibility in your back.

1 Kneel on the floor on your hands and knees with your hands positioned under your shoulders and your knees under your hips. Look straight ahead.

2 As you inhale, bring your chin up as far as is comfortable and arch your back downwards so the tailbone moves up.

3 As you exhale, tuck your chin into your chest and reverse the movement in your back so that your pelvis moves inwards, arching your back up.

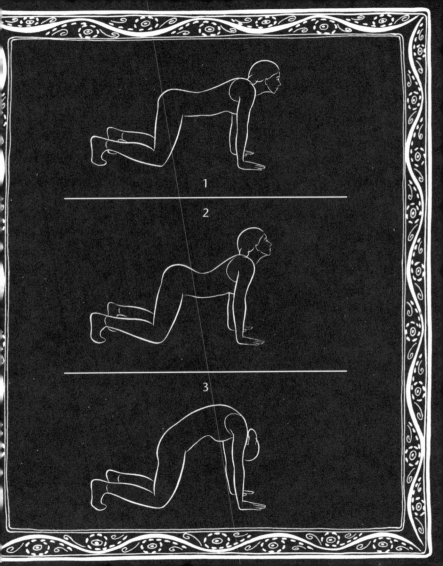

This simple hamstring stretch will help prepare your body for the more complex body stretch of Healing Tibetan Five.

Take Care

Hamstrings are easily strained; do not stretch further than is comfortable for you.

1   Sit on the floor with your legs together and your toes pointing up. Rest your hands on your thighs. Look straight ahead at your toes.

2   Keeping your eyes on your toes, bend over at the stomach, sliding your hands down your legs as far as is comfortable. Hold that position for ten seconds.

Slide your hands back up your legs as you straighten your spine and return to the start position.

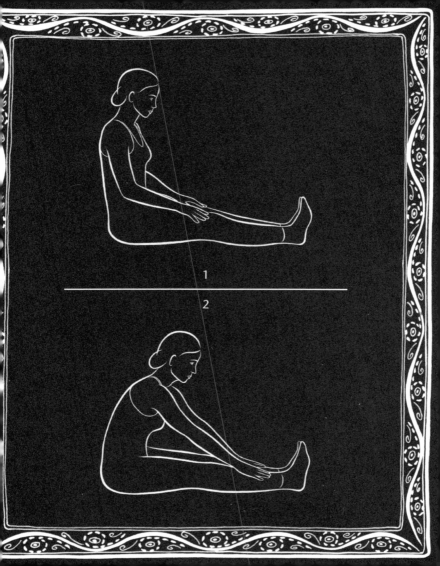

1

2

The Five
Healing Tibetans

Most people can start performing each of the exercises with three repetitions and, after a week or two, can increase the repetitions by three until each exercise involves 21 repetitions. (In general, 21 repetitions are enough to get the full benefit of each exercise.)

It doesn't matter how long it takes to build up to this number, but it is important that each exercise is performed correctly and smoothly without any need to rest between repetitions. Always do the same amount of repetitions for each exercise and, if at all possible, perform them every day.

Apart from Healing Tibetan Five, after each exercise stand straight with your arms relaxed by your sides and your eyes closed. Take two to three deep breaths before moving on to the next exercise.

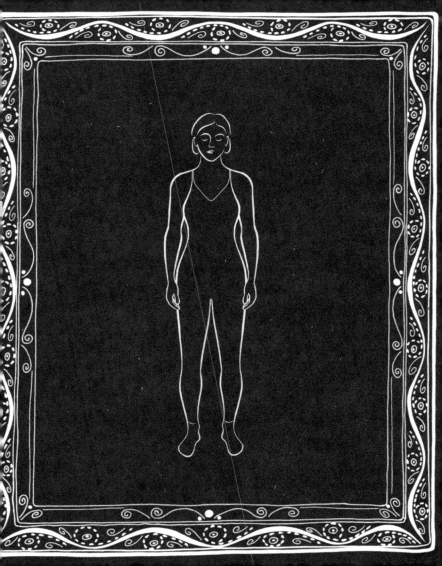

Healing Tibetan One

Among its other benefits, this exercise should help improve your sense of balance. Allow your sense of balance to develop naturally and do not use tricks to prevent dizziness (such as maintaining your focus on one point while spinning).

Take Care

Don't be tempted to spin too fast or you may fall over or move from the spot on which you should be spinning. It is best to start off slowly and increase the speed gradually. However, never spin so fast that you find it difficult to remain in one place while you spin.

1 Stand straight with your shoulders level and feet slightly apart. Hold your arms outstretched to the side at shoulder height with your palms facing downwards and your fingers and thumbs together. Face directly forwards. Begin breathing deeply and evenly.

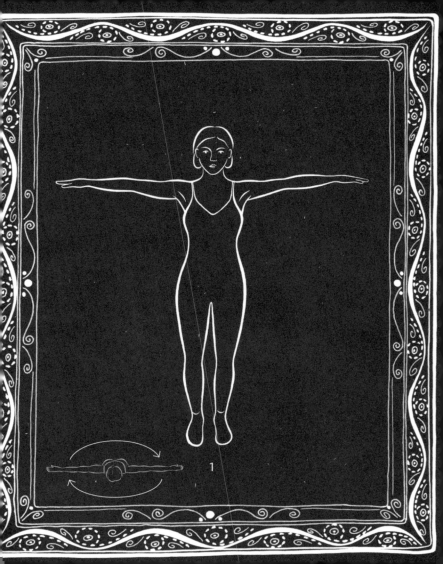

1

2   Keeping this position and still breathing deeply, turn on the spot to your right until you complete one full turn and you face the same direction as you started. Turn by taking small steps, leading with your right foot and following with your left foot.

Repeat three to four times at first, gradually building up to the full 21. (Do not pause between repetitions.)

Once you have completed the exercise, stand in the end position shown on page 33, breathing until any feelings of dizziness have subsided.

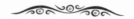

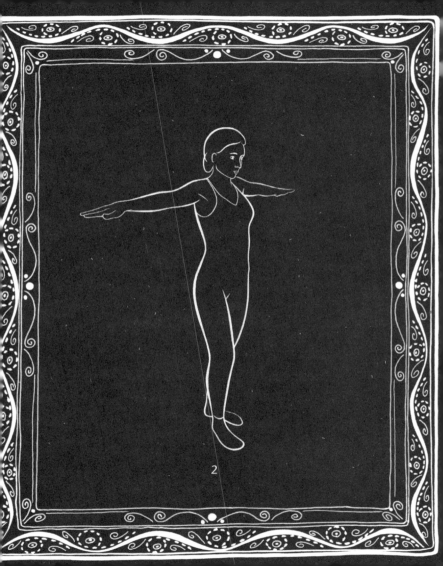

2

Healing Tibetan Two

Performing this exercise will strengthen your stomach muscles and, to a lesser extent, stretch your back.

Take Care

When you first perform this exercise, you may find you can do several repetitions with relative ease. However, do not allow this to deceive you into increasing the number of repetitions you do too quickly in case you injure the muscles in your stomach or back. Although pulled muscles will heal, it is better to progress more slowly and be confident you will not unduly strain your body.

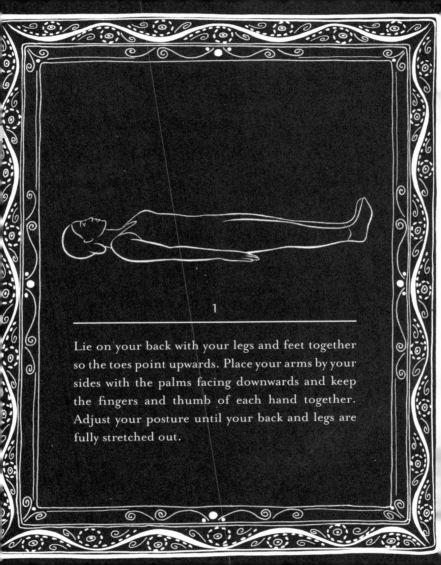

1

Lie on your back with your legs and feet together
so the toes point upwards. Place your arms by your
sides with the palms facing downwards and keep
the fingers and thumb of each hand together.
Adjust your posture until your back and legs are
fully stretched out.

2   Take a deep breath in, and as you inhale raise your head and your legs from the ground until your chin rests on or near your chest and your legs are completely vertical. When you are lifting your legs keep them together and as straight as you can, with your feet still touching. Avoid lifting your lower back off the ground: only your bottom should lift off the floor.

As you breathe out, lower your head and your legs to the ground until you return to the starting position. Make sure you raise and lower your head and your legs at the same speed.

Once you have completed the correct number of repetitions of this exercise, stand in the end position taking two to three breaths, then move on to Healing Tibetan Three.

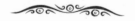

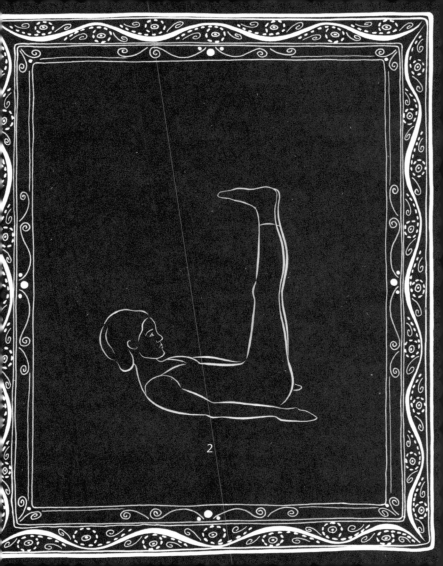

2

Healing Tibetan Three

The primary purpose of this exercise is to stretch your back and improve its flexibility.

Take Care

As with any exercise involving significant back movements, move slowly and smoothly and be careful not to overextend yourself.

I Kneel with your upper legs perpendicular to the floor, your legs slightly apart and your flexed toes on the floor. Your arms should be unbent and positioned by your sides. Hold your upper body upright, with your neck bent so your chin rests on or near your chest.

   (Alternatively, you can put the top part of each foot and its toes flat against the ground. Although this should improve how you arch your back, you may find it extends your ankles in a way that makes the exercise harder.)

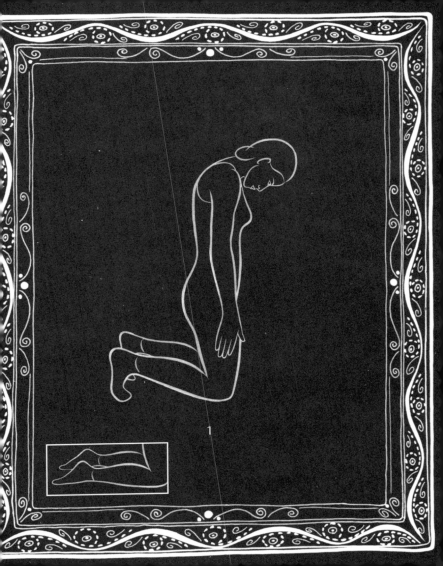

1

2   Breathing in, whilst keeping your upper legs perpendicular to the floor and your hands and arms still, lift your head and continue moving it until it is tilted as far back as is comfortable. At the same time, extend your spine backwards until you are bent as far back as you can manage. Initially, you may need to provide support with your hands during the backwards bend to avoid falling over and to keep your upper legs in position. However, after some practice you will find you can rely on the tension of the muscles in the upper legs and will no longer need to use your hands.

As you breathe out, move your head forwards and down, bringing your spine upright so that you return to the starting posture.

After the correct number of repetitions, return to the starting position (page 33) for a few moments.

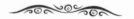

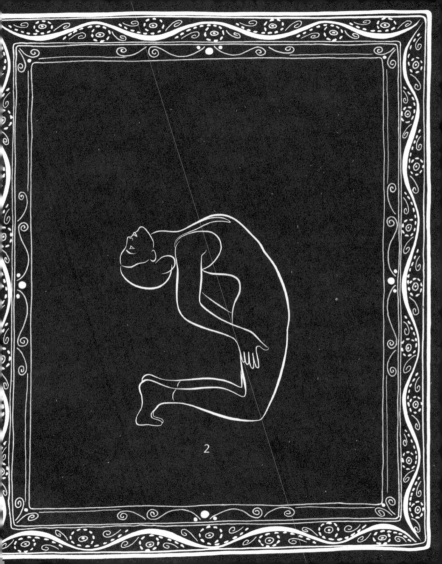

2

Healing Tibetan Four

This exercise helps build and maintain upper body strength.

Take Care

Supporting your upper body on your hands, palms down against the ground, can put stress on the wrists. If this is a problem, support your upper body with your hands formed into fists so the parts from the knuckles to the first finger joints touch the floor.

1   Sit on the ground with your legs stretched out in front of you and slightly apart so your feet and toes point upwards, in line with your shoulders. With your arms perpendicular to the ground place your hands palms down on the floor pointing towards your feet. Keep the fingers and thumb of each hand together. Bend your head forward so your chin rests on or near your chest.

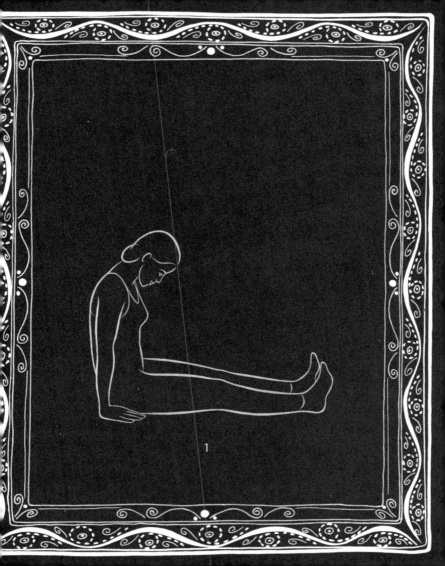

1

2   As you breathe in, lift your head until it is tilted as far back as is comfortable. At the same time, move your hips up and forwards until your torso is parallel to the ground and your lower legs are perpendicular to it.

Now breathe out, moving your head forwards and towards your chest, lowering your hips back towards the ground so you return to the starting position. Do not move your arms or hands, or allow your feet to slide during this exercise. Instead, pivot the motion of your upper body around your shoulders and the motion of your lower body around your ankles.

Don't forget to return to the standing position before moving on to the final exercise.

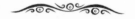

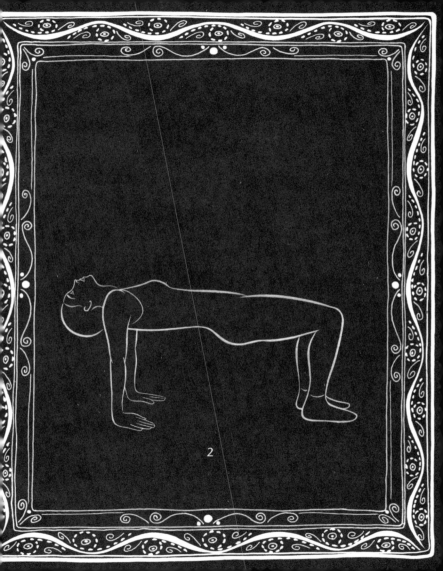

2

Healing Tibetan Five

The final position of this exercise involves a full body stretch, building on the different partial stretches involved in the previous exercises to improve your overall flexibility.

Take Care

Your arms and your legs should remain straight throughout; do not move your hands, or allow your feet to slide.

1   Lie on your front, but arch your upper body and head away from the floor. Flex your toes forward and keep your arms perpendicular to the ground, with your hands pointing forwards. Support yourself off the floor with just the palms of your hands and the base of your toes. Keep the fingers and thumb of each hand together. Tilt your head as far back as is comfortable.

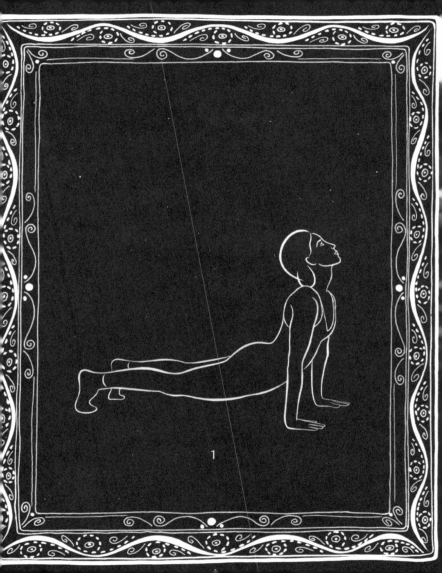

1

2   Breathing in, bring your head forward and your chin towards your chest. At the same time, move your hips up and back and your shoulders down and back so your lower body slants upwards and your upper body slants down until the whole body forms a reversed 'V'. If possible, have the soles of your feet touching the ground by getting your heels as close to the floor as you can. Although this may be hard to do at first, you should find angling your feet back from your toes in the starting position helps.

As you breathe out, lift your head away from your chest, lowering your hips towards the ground while raising your shoulders so that you return to the starting position.

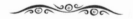

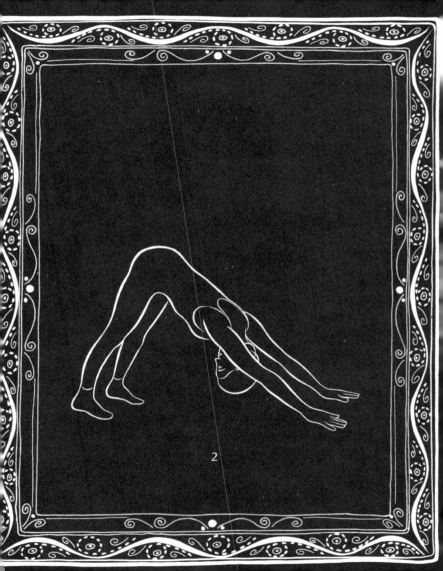

2

Healing Tibetan Six

Although this exercise accompanies the Five Healing Tibetans, and thus in some sense is a Sixth Healing Tibetan, it is not necessary to perform it to get the full benefit of the Five Healing Tibetans. The exercise has an energizing effect that is different to that of the other exercises and therefore is complementary.

Peter Kelder related this exercise to the raising of energy from lower energy centres in the energy body (see page 6) and suggested that only the celibate should perform it. However, this suggestion has more to do with the customs of the time he was writing in rather than any requirement of the exercise itself.

I Stand up straight with your arms by your sides and your feet slightly apart. Take a deep breath.

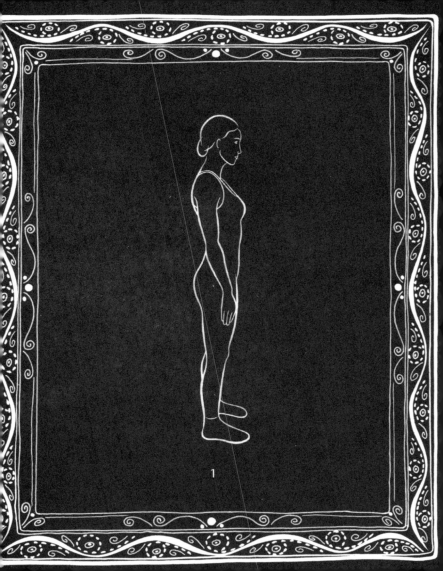

1

2 As you breathe out, bend your knees slightly and bend forward until you support your torso with your hands placed on your knees and your arms straight. Continue to breathe out, pressing in with the muscles of the lower abdomen first and then of progressively higher regions to force out all the air you can, until you can no longer breathe out.

3 Without breathing in, return to an erect position with your hands placed on your hips and your shoulders raised. Keep your abdomen pulled in and your chest pushed out. When you can no longer hold your breath, breathe in as deeply as you can through your nose. Then breathe out and return your arms to your sides.

Repeat the exercise no more than three times even if you do more repetitions for the five exercises that precede this one.

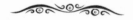

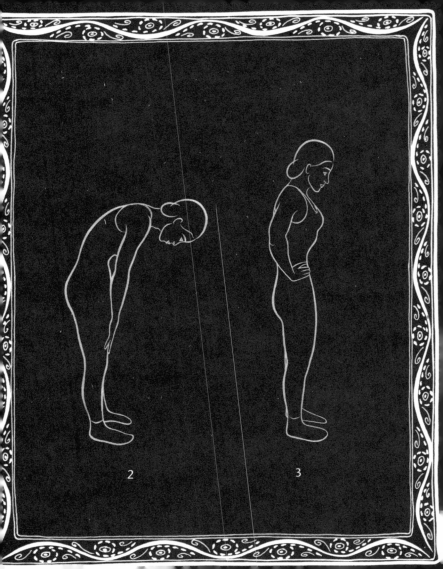

2

3

Meditations for the Five Healing Tibetans

The following meditations complement practice of the Five Healing Tibetans by helping to improve the health of your energy body.

The meditations are divided into two parts. The Nine Purifying Breaths dispel impurities from the energy body, and the visualization on page 62 reinforces the proper flow of energy throughout the energy body. Each part may be practised separately, but it is best to follow the order shown here.

Nine Purifying Breaths

Sit up straight with your legs crossed and your hands resting palm upwards in your lap.

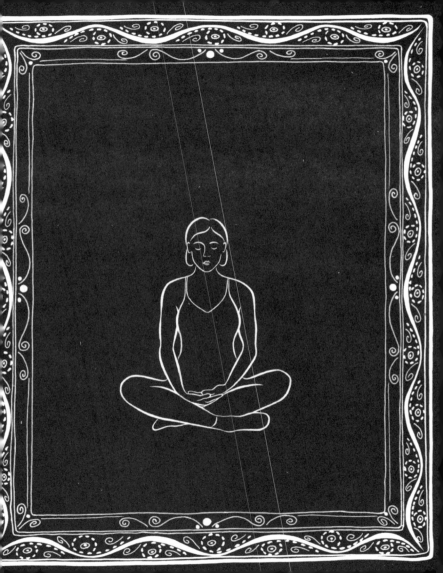

1   Keeping your right hand palm upwards on your right knee, turn your head to the right and press your left nostril shut with the index finger of your left hand, curling the other fingers and the thumb inwards. As you breathe in visualize that you inhale white light from your surroundings.

2   Before you exhale, rest your left hand palm upwards on your left knee and, turning your head to the left, press your right nostril closed with the index finger of your right hand. As you breathe out visualize that you exhale impurities from your energy body as black air. Repeat three times.

    Repeat for another three breaths, but switch the nostril of inhalation and the nostril of exhalation.

Return to the starting position with your hands folded palm upwards in your lap. Breathe in and breathe out through both nostrils. Visualize driving out the impurities from the top of your head when breathing out. Repeat twice more.

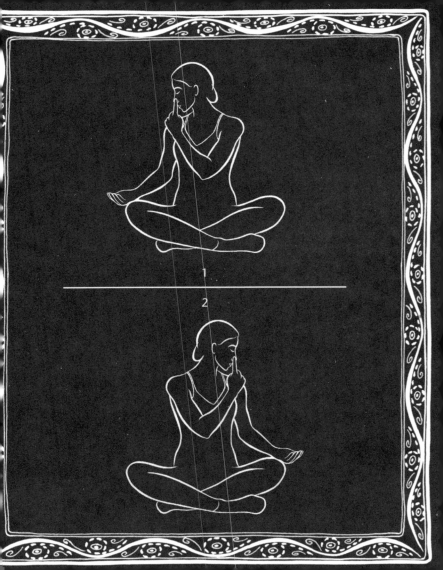

1

2

Visualization of the Energy Body

The second meditation is a visualization exercise. This meditation involves five chakras rather than seven so that you can focus on the differences in the energies of each chakra. (The energies of the top two are closely allied, as are the energies of the bottom two.)

Starting with your brow, focus on each of your energy centres in turn, singing OM for the brow, AH for the throat, HUM for the heart, SWA for the navel, and HA for the genital energy centre. Visualize each energy centre radiant with light: white for the brow, red for the throat, blue for the heart, yellow for the navel and green for the genital energy centre. Finally, visualize the central channel as a blue column uniting all the energy centres.

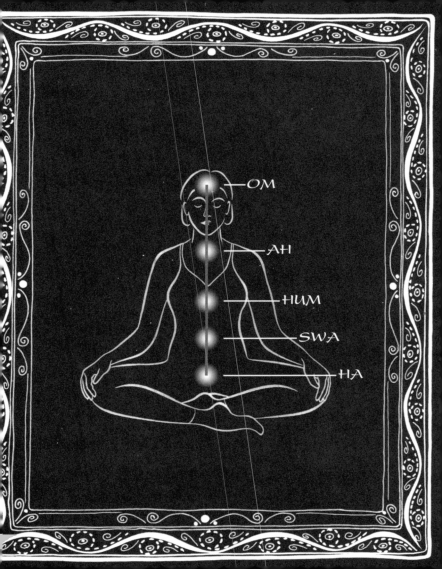